spOIL
Me

essentially speaking

Alysa Beer

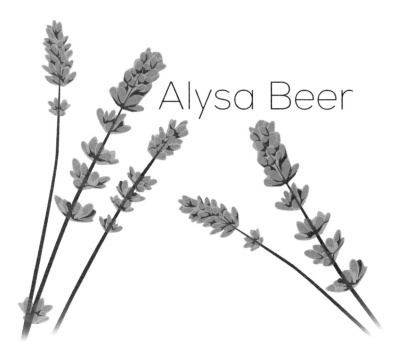

A POST HILL PRESS BOOK

spOIL Me
essentially speaking
© 2018 by Alysa Beer
All Rights Reserved

ISBN: 978-1-68261-741-0
ISBN (eBook): 978-1-68261-742-7

PRESS
posthillpress.com
New York • Nashville
Published in the United States of America

contents

revelations

my story

sometimes life overwhelms
kicks our knees right out from under us
blocks us
tries to prevent us from seeing what's good
from appreciating
how lucky we are
how truly blessed
beyond all else
glancing over at those we love
smiling, welling up
beaming with pride
all that they've accomplished
all that they've become
peeking into their futures
imagining
wondering
then all at once
the media slams
slams down hard
grabbing us tightly by the arms
yanking us
back to reality
slammed
the missing child
the sick friend
the corrupt politician
terrorism
drug addiction

mental illness
school shootings
pollution
the list eternal
yet close at heart
i know them
i feel their pain
my empathic nature
swallows me
i try to settle
as my heartbeat quickens
breath shortens
the knot twists and aches in my belly
the fears grip
taking over
the worries concern
perturb
disturb me
my oils serve me
they even my breathing
they untie my knots
offer innocence
purity, relief
they call me
with open arms
scents wafting as i unzip my bags
"my bags of magic potions," i tell my students
liberating
freeing
allowing me to think clearly
unobscured
removing emotion

erasing what looms
what lurks in dark corners
changing the way i live each day
how i view the world
its natural beauty and all that it offers
my oils do this
they allow me
lead me down a path of goodness
sureness, pureness
they ground me
offer direction
perfection
oils, dare i mention,
you spoil me!

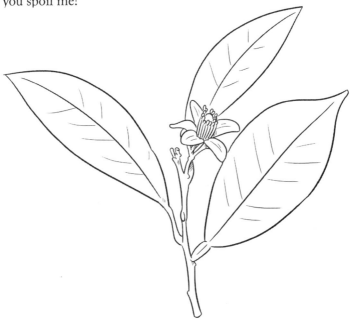

kari's story

she is nearly two years,
six months into her treatment
weak,
her body weak with stress
exhaustion, lack of sleep
pain, hunger, screams
no desire to eat
muscles breaking down
sickness abounds
it surrounds
lurks and lingers like a heavy rain cloud
about to burst
heaviness, worry
why isn't she eating?
why can't she keep anything down?
elevated levels
too high,
toxic
ammonia levels are toxic
need to feed her
not impede her
her body
unable to defend
reaching and grabbing
pulling and yanking at the feeding tube
vomit,
uncontrollable,
unstoppable
what to do?

doctors whispered
next steps
induce a coma
to steady her,
feed her,
to intubate,
make her whole again
something to get her back
back to being able to tolerate
such turmoil
complete and utter turmoil
nothing's working,
a thought surges
mind swirls
worry consumes
suddenly,
an epiphany
"god spoke to me"
literally
oils
should we try an oil?
we have dabbled here and there,
never truly understanding their power
can't deny, let's give it a try
time stands still
as she inhales
deeply and fully
filling her lungs and weakened body
deeply and fully
we watch as her face,
it brightens, it lightens
appetite heightens

then she speaks,
like an angel,
"spaghetti and french fries"
relief
much-needed comic relief
exchanging glances
analyzing circumstances
what were the chances?
certified pure therapeutic grade oils
we believe
could not conceive of their strength
power to heal
to reveal
the goodness of her body
inundated with chemical warfare
to eradicate the disease
this battle will be won
essentially stunned
new beginnings
chin up high,
move ahead
tears shed,
the joyous kind
blessings,
my blessings
oily, "pepperminty" essential oils,
you spoil!

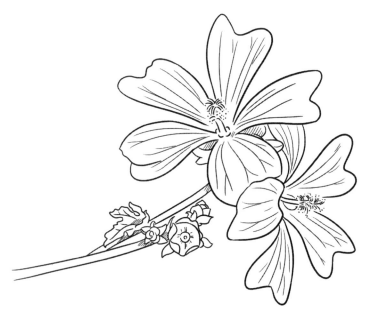

sheira's story

constipation
flatulation
medication
aggravation
stomach pain
belly protrusion
nothing helps
a foregone conclusion
digestive issues cause despair
seeking help everywhere
laxatives and pills to soften

overused,
all too often
sought out ways
to activate
educate
hoping to find relief
however brief
fennel oil
easing healthy digestion
she tried with no question
rubbed directly
on the belly
conducting movement
much improvement
a licorice-like flavor
life saver
game changer
offering relief
after years of grief
the seeds of the fennel plant
steam distilled to perfection
goodbye inflammation
discomfort abandoned
a new way of life granted
essentially grateful—oils,
you've spoiled!

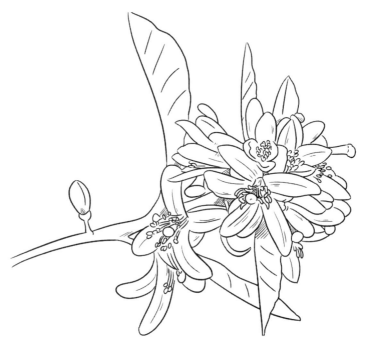

adrienne's story

it's time
flowing into life
the pain of birth
onto this earth
then flatline
stagnant air
cannot breathe
cannot move
waiting on angels' wings

all 7 of you
imprinted on my heart
etched in my memory
loss becomes triumph
creating family
building community
keeping connection
self-care
story shared
vulnerability shed
tears dried
gained perspective
ready to heal
faced reality
life renewed
aroma caught
oil's smells dispersed
hope restored
essence blended, creating hope
flowing
pouring open
eeceiving
inhaling life
newness
breathing in
living!

your story

distraction
inattention
inability to sit still
to follow direction
hyperactivity
impulsivity
never ceasing
never calm
the motor runs
twisting
turning
standing
sitting
cannot settle
disheveled
lack of organization
agitation
attentional challenges
baffle
frustrate
parents struggle
what to do?
who can help?
avoiding medication
negative relations
no one understands
can't meet demands
weight loss
moodiness

delayed growth
lack of sleep
is it worth risking?
need assistance
oils, can you help?
help to lull
to dull
the distractions
achieve satisfaction
enhance your focus
it's not hopeless
hoist attention
move in the right direction
a focus blend of oils is essential
in reaching one's potential
roll on the bottoms of the feet
temples, back of neck
on task? check!
note improvement
less movement
concentration
positive affirmation
a non-medical approach
a tough topic to broach
why not try?
one can't deny
this essential decision
is important to make
so much at stake
an oily endeavor
an organic pleasure
one that's treasured!

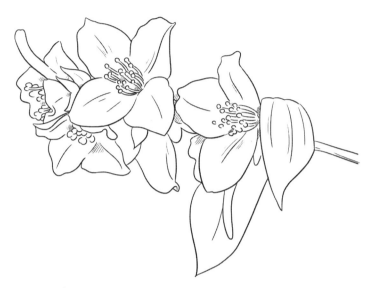

janet's story

she was nervous about the trip—
nervous to be on her feet all day long
walking cobblestone streets
pained
stabbing pain as she arose each day,
unable to find relief
stopping her
preventing her
getting in the way of her day-to-day
plantar fasciitis; chronic heel pain
wintergreen and spearmint oils are analgesic
these calm,
reduce pain,

and inflammation
enable movement
flexibility
ease into motion
one step at a time
massaging deeply
into her heel
over and over
again and again
sighs of relief
signs of healing
opportunities avail
essential to living an active life
filled with stories
firsthand experiences
shared with others
new beginnings
no stopping her,
nothing in her way
moving ahead,
for the first time,
in a long while
a healthier lifestyle
beguiled,
oils, you have spoiled
pain is foiled
yet again!

theresa's story

numbing, throbbing, cold
can't hold
anything
tips of fingers, weak and white
white, cold, numb fingers
limited circulation
discoloration, frustration
hidden
behind my gloves
gloves to protect
aching fingertips
tips that can't grip,
can't understand
can't bear—bare hands
humiliating,
insults berating
i'm a little girl wearing gloves at the pool
don't befool, so cruel, at school
harassed,
outcast,
picked last
self-esteem flounders,
no one around me
loneliness
raynaud's disease
someone said oils,
oils that navigate
can't wait

twist of fate
cypress oil,
you clear—
improve circulation
pure elation
blood flows
color grows,
no more whiteness,
not cold and lifeless
flexibility, dexterity
i'm back
it's me
renewed
exposure, closure
cypress oil, you spoil!

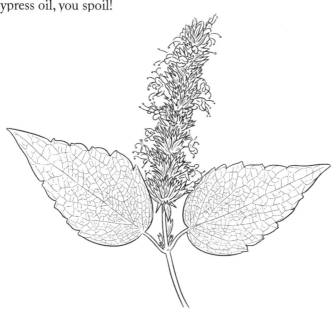

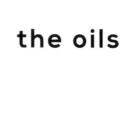

the oils

lavender

my bottles
they fix me
they lift me
empower me to heal
to educate
to heighten awareness of the body and mind
to soothe my soul and maintain balance
the balance to fight disease,
the balance to live my life in peace
without masking the pain,
without ignoring symptoms
my oils
they spoil
they piece together my loose ends and annihilate toxins
what ails you?
what presses upon you in the black of night?
mind racing, heart pounding, unforgiving,
unrelenting
heavy on my chest.
the world weighs on me.
i cannot slip out from under it.
oils, come spoil me,
help unravel my inside out
anxiety
not again
i feel it
i know it well
all too well.
why must it do this?

why must it interfere?
i was good;
at least i thought i was.
the thoughts
they don't stop.
they swirl and whirr.
does anyone see?
why didn't i think of that?
why did i say that to him?
the "*whys*" swallow me.
i cannot breathe
panic-stricken
my palms drip,
my ears ring
butterflies flop in my belly
i can't stop it
it only stops me
no more meds
no more sessions,
discussions, or check-ins
no more disappointments
only options
i need options
the option to take my healing into my hands
to tackle the fear
the panic
lavender
my first oil
my first try
my spoiler
it's aromatic power
the power to calm

the power to alleviate
a drop on my wrists,
a dab behind the ears,
now i inhale
my body slows as it deepens and fills me
seeps into my bloodstream and finds its own way
it knows what to do
it searches to repair what ails me.
inducing calmness and peace
i keep it close
close at all times
it serves me in so many ways.
when pressure outnumbers
when emotions skyrocket
lavender balances me,
levels me.

. . .

the sun makes me ache
ultraviolet heat burns
as i sit, as i wait,
irritates
fiery, red, raw,
lavender thaws,
it cools, it calms, it eases—
spoils me.

. . .

sleep
much-needed, never enough—
sleep
the clock ticks
time passes, light flashes
wandering mind, counting sheep
nothing
it was 1:00 now 2:00,
tomorrow lurks, so much to do
how will i cope?
questions reel
can't deal,
lavender
my blended lavender and coconut oil
i spritz my pillow,
mist my sheets
breathing in its magical scent,
i lay,
deep breath in—4 slow counts
out with 8—
i slow
tension releases from fingertips to toes
aware of my drifting
my falling,
digital numbers blur,
sounds fade
i sleep.
my blanket,
my lavender embraces me
spoils me

• • •

road trip
time to leave
they scurry away,
they hurry
they run, they hide
scared of the upcoming ride
what to do—
our furry friends need oils, too
a drop on the collar and back of the neck
lavender soothes
my anxious pets
calm sets in,
resistance goes
tension releases
restful feelings
comfort permeates
peace resonates
out the door, garage slams
alarm sounds
hope abounds
oils, you spoil
and salvage my sanity.

Alysa Beer

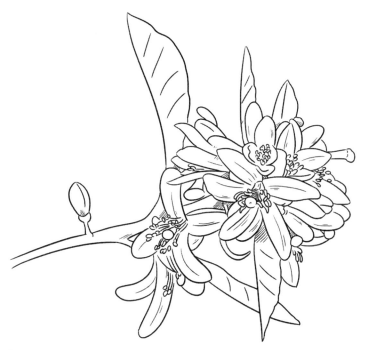

lemon

emotions. basic human emotions
why must they be so toxic?
toxicity
toxic relationships
toxic environments
toxic habits
toxicity clogs
it inhabits our cells, it clogs

can't breathe. swelling with negativity
my oils release, diffuse
clear thoughts
decisions made
to consider:
what we put in our bodies matters
medications are contaminants
they do their job and continue to destroy,
not knowing what is necessary
not knowing what is left
synthetic toxins.
unknowing.
essential oils know
they satisfy
they balance
they search for abnormalities
never ceasing until they're found
congestion
emotional and physical congestion
the bad breakup
you argued with your brother
the failing grade on the test
the feeling of rejection
my oils detoxify
they cleanse
breathe
spoil me, lemon oil
soak me in your citrus
freshness from your rind
our leading antimicrobial agent
destroying bacteria
antiseptic

immune-builder
germ-killer
bug-repeller,
pick-me-up,
concentration, stimulation,
brain energy
one drop, just one
early morning drop in your water
natural cleansing, a carminative
acid reducer, digestive helper,
appetite suppressor,
antibacterial
lemon cleaner, throat soother,
taste enhancer.
lemon, you spoil me
your scent restores me.

• • •

my husband's baseball caps
dirty, grimy, baseball caps
stained with sweat
soaked and worn
pathogens airborne
never ceasing
odors releasing
lemon oil,
come spoil this scent
remove germs as you work your wonders
4 drops of lemon in your washing machine
soak, wash and spin

goodness from within
limonene from the rind
smells divine
hats disinfected
organically protected
purified
doubts subside
lemon oil, you've spoiled
yet one more time!

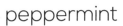

peppermint

herbs. peppermint herbs
(mentha piperita).
ancient medicine,
soothe muscles, open constrictions
dilution, massaged temples
tension,
tension headache,
soothe it, relax it,

pain relief
migraines
constricted vessels.
improve me,
its menthol decongests,
deepens breath
expectorant loosens, natural solutions
sinusitis, bronchitis,
peppermint oil, you spoil,
you rid my body of pain
stinging, clinging to me,
zinging, heightening my awareness
perk me up,
enhance my work
help me to burn the midnight oil
focus me, energize me
slow breath in,
repeat,
breathe
inhale again,
"mmmmm"
clears my airways, opening, relaxing,
eliminating pollen, allergies dissipate
peppermint, you cool, you heighten concentration at school,
stabilize a fever,
naturally,
organically
aspirin-free
with versatility, you're cherished
multi-faceted,
menthol, peppermint

• • •

the next day,
the early wake up
the bed spins, and stomach wrenches
what did i drink?
the wine? the espresso vodka shots?
pounding, throbbing head
pit in the stomach that won't forgive
what was i thinking?
trying to forget
forget what's hard
i wasn't thinking
peppermint oil
help me unfurl
help me calm the storm in my body
a drop on my thumb and quick to the roof of my mouth,
then 2 more on my hands and rub my belly,
a drop on my button, like the cherry on top
reapply, as needed, no waiting, no 6 hours till my next dose,
reapply
the oil seeps
deep
my certified pure therapeutic grade oils
100% fresh and distilled
from the plant leaf, resin, root
where it knows, knows to go
to heal me, to flush my body of what's unwanted

• • •

summer days, ocean breeze
mike's boat
couldn't wait, saved the date
ready to go
looks rough,
i consider,
rougher than i thought
rougher than he said
up, down, up, down
my stomach churns,
up, down, up, down
my insides burn
need cooling,
peppermint cooling
oil save me,
i'm losing my mind
up, down, up, down
some know the feeling
the waves are stealing
my goodness, my summer day
hold on tight
grab my bottle,
peppermint oil delights
ease my weakened limbs,
as we swim up high on the waves,
more peppermint oil i crave,
inhale in and then slow exhale out
once again, nausea abounds
2 drops on my tongue,
2 behind the ears,
its power
its strength

eyes shed tears
down my face. stop this,
balance me, oil, as my insides coil
tightness, contraction, need action
the menthol soothes, it moves me
body loosens, gives up
nausea passes,
eases,
dies.
another battle won
victorious
laborious peppermint
heaven sent!

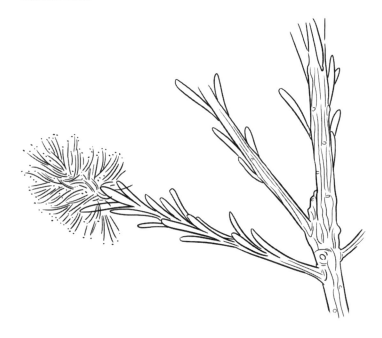

melaleuca

paper cut
tiny yet fierce
stinging, burning, unyielding
throbbing, pulsating, beating
in the bend of the finger,
in constant motion, gripping in pain
need protection to deter infection
melaleuca oil, a healer,
brings immediate relief, sheer disbelief
the green-head fly bite, mosquitoes nag
dab on site, as the healer heals
pain-redirecting, melaleuca's disinfecting
no mark, no scar, no spot remains
melaleuca cicatrizes, it neutralizes,
diminishes any signs, not a trace
clears away blemishes, any size.

• • •

lice
ancient nuisance
source of shame, anxiety and stress
unavoidable
but controllable
lice love humans
their scent, their warmth
lice swarm
tea tree oil (melaleuca) is essential here

lice despise that smell and *flee* in fear
(no pun intended)
2-3 drops gently combed through
it's strong flavor knows precisely what to do
an all-natural remedy to fight
this annoying parasite
be proactive with kids in school
2-3 drops regularly in your shampoo
lice, beware—
we're prepared
melaleuca oil in hand, don't despair.

• • •

hands shyly in pockets, slightly embarrassed
the skin-colored arrangement
circling my nail beds:
warts.
ugly, dry, peeling, infected
warts
manicure beware, contagious, infectious
barriers, boundaries, they stay away
melaleuca
spoil me, oil!
do your thing
fix me,
i douse with oil and cover tightly,
airtight
repeat, day-in, day-out
one by one, they open,
wounds open

dry, peel away, disappear
relief, clearing,
no one's even staring,
i'm free,
free to wave hello,
free to shake your hand
melaleuca, stay close
i'll share you, share your goodness
share your healing power,
but my bottles run out,
they empty from use
treasures lost,
only to be found again
swaddled in bubble wrap,
delivered with grace
happiness is the ring of my doorbell,
my package,
my gold,
my treasure,
my oils
i'm spoiled

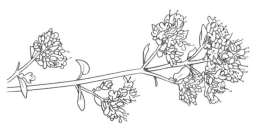

oregano

there's a fungus among us—
of the toe—
more common than most know
no friend, but foe,
essential oregano
the pizza oil, its smell
so potently fills a room
mountain-grown, abundantly known
protects
fights bacterial infection, cold and flu
immune system booster, antifungal
emmenagogue,
sore throat improver
ear infection soother
this oil is "hot"
sensitive on the skin,
so please dilute
one can't refute
it's power to ward off toxins
is absolute
oregano oil

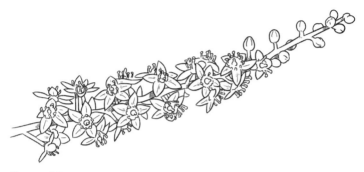

frankincense

disease
always lurking
who is next—
who will be the next victim?
add one more name
to the list of many
friends and family,
young and old
disease doesn't discriminate
it takes
it dehumanizes
dehumanizes the mind, the body, the heart
fear
fear of its fierce return
when will it be back?
i know it will
tests
the worry every time, sleepless nights
helpless, hopeless,

fingers crossed, prayers spoken
bodies are weakened, cells disoriented,
imbalance, toxic imbalance
vulnerability
disease strikes, cells confused
inflammation, abnormal cells configure
need to break through, need redirection
frankincense oil
the leader, the fighter, the destroyer
knows the body
claims the good and combats the bad
leaves healthy cells strong
diminishes cells that have gone awry
researchers search
discoveries unearthed
pray for a cure
frankincense: integrity, honesty, pure
an ancient cure
my go-to, every day.
i matter,
my family matters
empowerment
meaningful empowerment
taking our health and wellness in our own two hands
seeking prevention,
this search motivates us
changes us for the better
to balance our bodies,
to steady our emotions
homeostasis
eliminating vulnerability
limiting attacks

attacks of the body and mind
steadying,
regularity,
reducing the chemicals we put in our bodies
choosing organically,
cleansing,
purifying
from the earth
from the tree
from the leaf
the resin
the root
the petal
the flower
distilled to perfection
essentially an extension of me
my oils
they spoil me
completely.

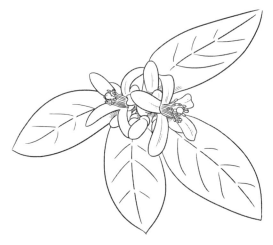

grapefruit

diet
need to lose
just a few,
clothes feel snug
need an extra tug
to get my jeans past my hips
tight in the waist
it frustrates
diets
tried them all
frustrated
despised,
diets
grapefruit—certified pure therapeutic grade
extracted straight from the rind

promotes a healthy metabolism
tastes divine
one to two drops in my water
i swish around each day
eliminating sugar cravings
pounds drop, drop away
no urges, no desires
slowly, surely, i sip my grapefruity potion
energy rises, invigorates
clarifies, motivates
grapefruit oil, you spoil
helping to achieve,
with ease
more productive,
less disruptive
your flavor erupts
awakens taste buds
cravings simplify,
can't justify
not having you around
close by, within my reach
i preach, sharing the wonder
"you should try," i often say
grateful to give it away
to share its goodness, its power
its ability to change lives
grapefruit oil, you've changed me
delicate yet deliberate
you've changed me
you spoil, grapefruit oil!

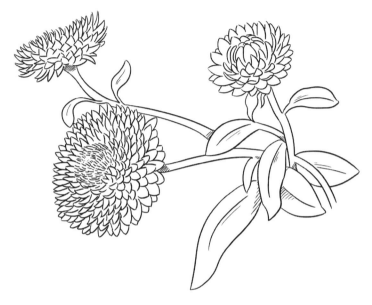

helichrysum

oil of the greek gods
native to the mediterranean region
"helios" means sun, and "chrysos" is gold
beautiful golden sunshiny flower
endless benefits, extreme power
optimizes heart health
and respiratory unrest
heals the skin, anti-aging
uv light protector, acne aiding

may reduce kidney stones
by detoxifying the unknowns
helps to reduce bloating,
a natural diuretic
empathetic
gut healer
natural glow revealer
helichrysum oil,
you spoil

respiratory blend

asthma,
it frightens,
airways tighten
the stress of not knowing
sheer distress,
no air flowing
inhaler by my side,
waiting,
waiting for constriction
from allergens that lurk
feline dander, hay fever unfolds
pollens, grasses, spores of mold
breathing worsens, heavies
oils help me steady
steady my breathing as i inhale their power
eucalyptus, peppermint, cardamom, ravintsara,

clear my swelling passages
calm my wheezing,
coughing, sneezing
control my symptoms naturally,
chemical-free
no toxins, just purity
my oils, you spoil me

vetiver

evening sets in
my day closes
it's done
time to retreat
to deplete
that last bit of strength
used in a day
i lay
considering what my body needs
what potion shall i concoct
drop by drop?
pondering emotions
feeling what my body might need
to free
what lingers?
A vine of today's mishaps
wraps me tightly

regrets, perhaps
need grounding
finding
vetiver root
a hearty grass oil
vertically grown
grows deeply into soil
rooting its way
down
sturdily, robustly,
deeply trusting
grounding me
steadying my uneasiness
diffusing continuously
as sleep comes,
her warm embrace,
thoughts erased
prepared to face
what life serves
vetiver, you preserve
balance conserved
reserved just for me
essentially spoiled, indeed

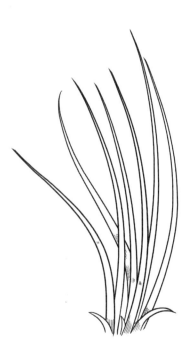

classroom blues

a cough,
a sniffle,
an itch,
hocking, spittle,
sinus drip,
ooey gooey germs
sickness confirmed
strep, fevers, stomach bug
over-the-counter and prescription drugs
Why not defend, prepare, and act?
energizing our immune systems upon contact
clove bud, cinnamon leaf, eucalyptus and rosemary
oils that fight off germs; extraordinary
a spritz in my classroom
to purify the air
can energize too, if diffused
a drop on my tongue
or in my water each day
immune-boosting power
direct from the flower
this blend of oils spoils.
protects us
naturally
organically.

essential inspirations

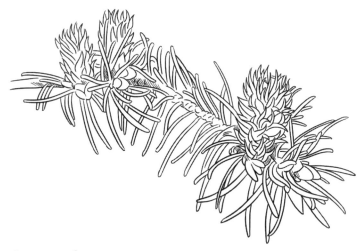

the scent of a rose
is its essence,
hence, it's essential oil

how do you do it all, oils?
how can you be all of those things to all of us?
you promote clarity of thought
banish my mental fatigue
i use your power
your power to reason, to solve problems calmly
to raise awareness, to take healing in my own hands
empowerment oils,
you empower me!

i am not a salesperson,
i am a sharesperson

my oils balance me
they prevent me from shattering,
but they aren't shatterproof,
no, not at all
nothing is perfect.

some say the best way to receive an oil's goodness is through
inhalation
2 drops in the palm of your hand
rub your palms together
open them ever so slightly
poke your nose within
deep breath in
as the oil vaporizes
as it enters nasal passages
causing sensations that can surprise
then slowly breathe out
repeat several times
inhalation = 100% satisfaction

life isn't perfect because of my oils
life is perfect because i have tools
my oils are my tools
they give me options
i can choose how to tackle this or that,
rather than popping a pill or calling a doctor
oils, you spoil me!

essential oils are funny
unpredictable and smart
because our bodies get bogged down
stress, toxic thoughts, congestion
too much to mention
oils help our bodies
to do what our bodies needs to do
because it just can't do it at the moment
funny to imagine
that our bodies can't figure it out
we offer our bodies help
we offer our bodies the essentials it needs to work in balance
homeostatically
perfectly
productively
this is when the oils spoil
they fix what's clogged,
congested, infected
physical wellness
emotional wellness
why wouldn't you try—
attempt to help your body work
work in the way nature meant it to?
oils are working,
inside the body
sometimes unrecognizably
always sizably
trust it,
believe
allow yourself to accept
the gifts
the pure and essential gifts
that oils have to bestow.

oils aren't magic, not a panacea or a quick fix
essential oils are an education; a movement
not to be taken lightly
a force to be reckoned with
learn with me!

when people say, "there's an oil for that"
they don't always know what it is.
there's an honesty that comes with our oils
there's a community that comes with our oils
everything related to our oils is goodness and because of that,
the answer always appears.

my oils unstick me
they keep me on my toes and alert
there's no giving up when you have essential oils as a resource
The only limit is not giving them a chance
when you shut them down
when you don't believe they can help
that is when you stop yourself before even trying

i'm a wellness advocate
because i believe in these oils
because i believe in their innate power
the power to do in my body what is needed
to make me wholesome and healthy
to keep me strong enough
to weather any storm
i choose wellness
i'm a wellness advocate.

no one oil does one thing
that would be too easy
there's nothing easy about essential oils
they are complex

new oil discoveries happening all the time
breakthroughs in medical treatments
shocking improvements to our emotional and physical health
that's why i can't live without them

purity is critical
quality is key
don't be fooled by oils you meet along the way
purity is pivotal
without it, benefits are limited
with it, benefits are limitless.

essential oils contain no fatty acids
making them non-oily
these oils are simply not oil
isn't that weird?

i treasure using my oils each day
Because i remember my days without them
when my struggle was real
when my head pounded relentlessly
no more pain relief could be found
until i found my oils
i was restricted
now i am boundless!

most of what i receive from my oils
is the joy i get when discovering they help others
there's nothing better than seeing that look
the look of relief when one is unburdened from pain
there's nothing better than hearing that sound
the sound of her voice as she thanks me for her oils
these are the joys of essential oils

i massaged my aunt's toes
toes scarred with surgery
scarred with age
scarred with pain
i rubbed my oils in and around them
feeling their coldness warm
feeling their hardness soften
seeing the wince of affliction dissipate
this is why i do what i do;
these are the moments that matter

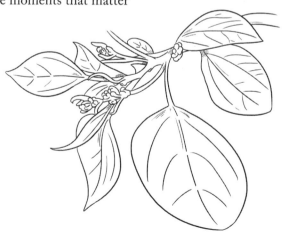

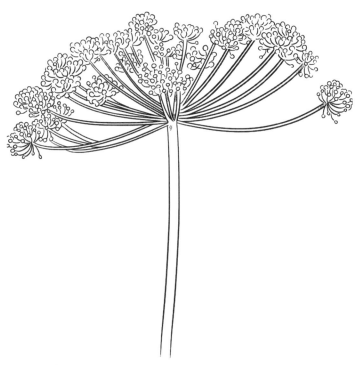

nerve pain
neuropathy
peripheral neuropathy
caused by diabetes or nerve damage
hard to manage
never ceasing
or decreasing
aching, pain
numbness, tingling
muscle spasms
need an inkling

a glimmer
an ounce
of hope
of help
to stop it
to quiet its harshness
marjoram oil, come spoil
analgesic, anti-spasmodic nerve tonic
these feelings are chronic
help me cope with my symptoms
increase circulation
right on location
never stop searching
continuous urging
be resourceful
forceful
seek out alternatives
to soothe and treat symptoms
don't be a victim
this is your life
this is your pain
combat it
healthfully, safely
oils are essential here,
nothing to fear!

i wish you'd believe me
have faith in what i say
we are programmed
(understandably so)
to negate what is natural and organic

we have become an impatient society
one seeking a "quick fix"
a bandage to affix, to hide
we must dig deeper
look in depth for answers,
solve the mysteries of our flaws
flaws that cause weakness and stress
discover the deeper reasons
rip away what is hiding
look what is before you
don't negate the answers
they exist
we grow from knowledge
do not fear the unknown
our routines stop us
block us from seeing what is new
prevent us from mending ourselves
discover the essential fixers, healers
oils
see with me
believe with me!

essential oils create harmony
harmony of mind, body and spirit

rethink your medicine cabinet with essential oils

our skin is our most underused organ
why not use it?

i'm tickled pink
as i watch you take an oil
i'm pleased
as you pick it up out of my bag
i'm humbled
to see you can benefit
i'm relieved
that it fits you
it eases your ache or burn
it calms as you discern
as you learn
learn to heal
to heal with oils.

here's an essential truth
one that may be new to you
essential oils can be categorized
after their chemistry is carefully analyzed
either calming or uplifting,
pick or choose
which do you need now?
which will you use?
florals are calming,
as are trees,
herbs, and grass oils
they offer grounding
calming
relaxing
while mint oils are known to energize
they are uplifting

good moods maximize
the sweetness of citrus
warmth of spice
inspire feelings of paradise
see—my oils—they're not easy
they inspire me to study, to seek
their history,
their chemistry
endless information
conversation
connection
possession
increasing my collection
emotional attachment
compassion, advancement
new studies are plentiful
more secrets unfurling
ideas whirling
you never cease to amaze me, oils
you are essential to me.

why oils? why choose oils? our world is bombarded with
industry. production. machinery. pollution. our air, our
water, polluted. soil soaks it up, drinks it. slurps its sludge,
its muck, its poison. never meant for us. but it's ours. part of
our everyday lives. as we breathe it, or eat it, or drink it. fast
food, artificially colored and flavored. chemically produced.
cleaning products, pesticides, deodorants; unnatural, toxic,
synthetic. we have become weak. sick. oils provide natural
solutions. plant based herbal therapy. mother nature's hand-
iwork. endless benefits that have been ours since the begin-

ning of time. right at our fingertips. accessible. how did we
let them get away? how did we let pharmaceuticals usurp our
innocence—displace what we knew to be right—what we
knew to be authentic? essential oils reconnect us. optimize
us. give us a healthier way of life. a life of purity. 100% pure
therapeutic grade oils, you definitely spoil us.

i step outside myself.
watching
in awe
since my oils and i first met
i've grown, calmed, balanced
i've discovered how to be,
to be at ease
feelings of impatience
seem less
digress
my body is contented
re-oriented, re-organized
it works easier
less turbulent
less roiled,
well-oiled
smoother
fitter
more wholesome
it's hard to imagine
what life was like
before my essentials were essential
they were inconsequential
today my oils inhabit my thoughts

my decisions, my discussions
all day, every day
always striving to share them
to spread their generosity
reciprocity
we are in this together, oils:
you and me

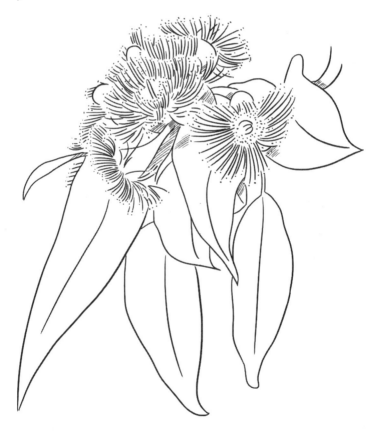

the truth is
using essential oils has transformed me
convinced me
helped me
to depend less on pharmaceutical intervention
more on intention
the intention to find alternatives
to treat day to day ailments more naturally
healthfully,
safely
helping others understand they have options
this has become my mission
quite an easy decision!

when i'm feeling down
no matter how much
when someone asks about oils,
my ears perk
my heart jerks
they clear me
they cheer me
to know that i can share
to repair
an aching heart,
sore muscles,
or body part
it's always a thrill when i can make a connection
for someone
my oils are there,
every minute of every day
for us all

to engage
to embrace
today is the day
to initiate
i'll begin with you,
to facilitate
to alleviate
to advocate
essential oils will spoil you too,
just you wait!

just because i love my oils
doesn't mean i'm naive
or delusional
their goodness is not an illusion
that only i believe
i don't need convincing
they work for me
they work for those around me
i believe in their power
in their goodness.

my oils are my favorite way
of optimizing a healthy way
of minimizing the number of toxins
i put in my body
minimizing the number of toxins
my family puts in their bodies
instead of popping a pill
i pop open my bottles and out pours
350 drops of concentrated goodness!

with change comes controversy,
with change comes resistance
with change comes adversity
too much to handle
creating scandal
please,
don't criticize me for taking my health into my own hands,
for finding success and wanting to share that with others
i'm not trying to scam or trick you into believing.
give oils a chance
try them out
see what you think
integrate them into your life
simply, truly, authentically, and genuinely
oils, they do spoil.

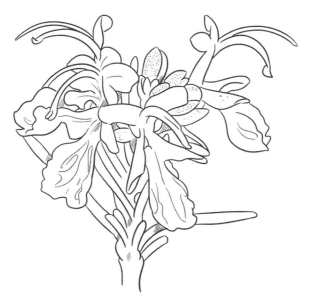

emphatically aromatic

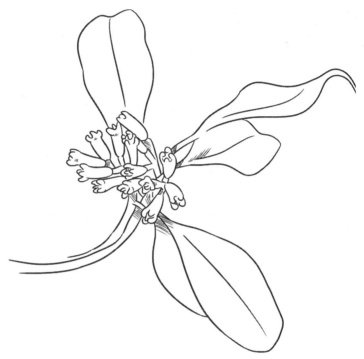

aromatherapy

an alternative to medicines
therapeutic grade oils, the purest
massaged in our bodies
infused in our baths
diffused in the air
inhaled
it's how we delight in our oils

how we choose
to make them personal
olfaction, our sense of smell
detects molecules in the air
making them essential
signaling the brain
our limbic system
controlling behaviors and emotions
memory formations
memories connect us
to our pasts
triggering old feelings
pumpkin pie in the oven
fresh-cut grass
we tell our stories
pass down our jewels
holding them closely
tucked away securely
until we are reminded again
olfaction,
molecules in action
pure satisfaction
these scents make no sense
yet, they have the power to transport us
take us back,
to another time
to another place
scents are triggers
emotional triggers
good and bad
happy and sad
scents make no sense.

grandma

i remember grandma's scent,
mothballs
"they keep the moths away, honey," she'd say
they were grandma
warm hugs, endless love,
playing cards, ice cream sundaes
mothballs

aromas

sweet-smelling oils
remind me of…
smell like…
the quickest way to affect our mood
is through our sense of smell

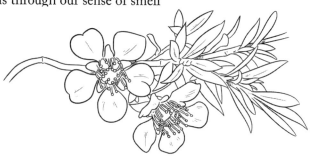

mrs. j.

mrs. j's gravy
you could almost taste it from down our street
the doors of the bus swung open
the smell lifted us
a magic carpet ride
over to mrs. j's
wednesdays were gravy days,
wednesdays were the best days
spaghetti, gravy, homework,
mrs. j and me

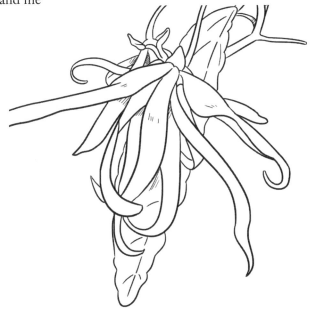

nanny

nanny's perfume
her signature scent
unmistakably hers,
lingers long after she goes
precedes her every arrival
undeniably hers
in an instant
in the midst of a crowded train station
that smell
i glance behind me
expecting her
over my shoulder
looking for her
ahead,
she's not there
her scent grabs me
envelops me in her warm hug
shakes me,
reminding me
transporting me
to the last time
her blue eyes haunt
her dentures click
her voice, i hear it
inside me
part of me
aromatic power
amazes and defies
our everyday expectations
keeps people close
in our hearts and minds.

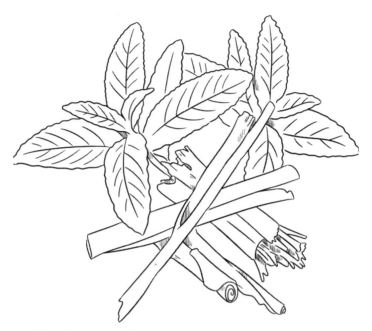

diffusingly infusing

diffusing
soothing
fills a room
aromatically pleasing
releasing, increasing
dodging pathogens,
before they invade,
uplifting mood,
changing attitude

attitude toward work
positivity
productivity
builds success
success in the workplace
success in our relationships
the power of diffusion
oil infusion.

tiny molecules

my oils
tiny molecules
leaping in the air
detected as smells
i open my bottles.
from across the room,
scents zoom
within minutes
know no limits
can't diminish
their power, their ability
causing volatility
excitement in me
tiny molecules
leaping in the air
oils, you spoil me.

sick

doctor says,
it's viral,
strength spirals
downward
i'm weak,
can't speak
throat's sore
abhor
can't ignore,
what to use,
to diffuse
choices
i have choices
pop the top
4 small drops
scent envelops
my room
my walls
my body
essential in my healing
essentially speaking,
my oils, they spoil.

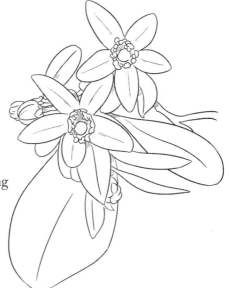

a year in oils

january

it's a new year,
setting resolutions,
requiring inner strength
and confidence
travelling down new paths
quest for adventure
cardamom oil builds open mindedness
and a hunger for new thoughts and ideas
tangerine oil helps us to accept change
and eliminates anxiety when doing so
letting go, releasing
resolving
now the celebration,
pop the cork,
choose confidence as you embark
on this new year, this new you
spoil yourself
feel compelled
their benefits are unparalleled

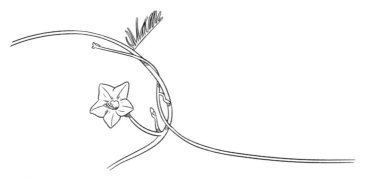

february

next month awaits,
a chill, a shiver,
warmth delivers
it's valentine's day
chocolates, flowers, romance surrounds
set the mood with oils,
their power resounds
creating an atmosphere
one that is alluring
reassuring for lovers
an aphrodisiac blend of oils
jasmine, wild orange, patchouli
enhancing sensuality
add sandalwood oil and ylang-ylang too
those oils know what to do
essentially for you
rose oil
farmed in bulgaria
pure therapeutic grade rose oil

252,000 individual petals
8,000 rose flowers,
1 bottle of rose oil
nothing says "i love you" better
rub on the neck and wrists
cannot resist
the fragrance it transmits
stirring romance
passion enhanced
entranced
rose oil, you spoil

valentine's day proposals,
or wedding night bliss,
neroli's orange blossom scent
pierces your heart and love augments
deeply intoxicating fragrance,
fosters radiance,
increases libido
awakens sexual interest
its flowery fragrance exploding with citrus
neroli oil
a true spoiler
inhibition destroyer
establishes enjoyment
poignant

march & april

easter and spring go hand in hand
budding trees, resurrection
grateful feelings, deep reflection
cleanse the body and mind
vibrant colors, all aligned
peel off the layers of insulation
joyous thoughts, essential inspiration
rebirth ignites positive intention
clary sage dropped in a warm bath
creates a more positive path
rub on the bottoms of the feet
directly on pulse points, to defeat
negative thoughts surrender
a true defender
spring's re-emergence
melissa oil
"the oil of light"
brightens and lifts
attitudes shift
dispels negativity
we know this with certainty
rubbed on forehead, shoulders or chest
lifts feelings, eliminates stress
easing us forward with revitalization
raising us up with elation

with this season comes realignment
spring cleaning, overhaul & consignment
emptying cupboards and closets
a job that's colossal
thyme oil removes dirt and grime
cleansing stains and sticky slime
sanitizing without noxious agents
remedies that are truly ancient
open the windows,
push open the door
diffusing these oils
splendor ignites
fennel seed oil
supports spring's transformation
improving productivity
and concentration
its molecules spring forth in the air
seeping into our bodies with comfort and care
spreading, detoxifying, filling
easing our transition
on a mission
help us to heal
with aromatic appeal
essentially attached
perfectly matched
oils spoiling
as we are enjoying
their every benefit.

may

may flowers burst
we feel a thirst
a hunger to be outside
in the open air
awnings are hoisted
porches are swept and uncovered
decorated
your presence requested
for the upcoming fiesta
it's cinco de mayo
essential recipes
oily specialties
using lime and cilantro oils to flavor dips and salsas
lemon oil, with avocado
guacamole aficionado
señor and señorita
would you like a margarita?
rosemary & wild orange oils
lend the perfect flavor
a mere extension of nature
raise your glass in celebration
"aceite esencial"
essential oils are a sensation

june

essential oils don't discriminate
father's day gifts for your mate
do it yourself, "diy"
a father's day surprise
a soothing cream for shaving
your hubby will be raving
add 5 drops of each oil
get ready to spoil
patchouli oil moisturizes
peppermint will cool
top it off with ginger
a spicy kick
easy and quick
sharpens the mind
memory refined
headache reliever
success achiever
the perfect blend
to honor him
oils, you spoil
again and again

school is out,
summer vacation
relaxation
outdoor play
possible travel
perfect time to dabble
to learn more about

this oil obsession
need in my possession
for summertime survival
their power's unrivaled
melaleuca or tea tree oil
essential bug repelling
camphor-smelling
calming rashes, cuts and gashes
killing germs
oils reaffirm
a must for the season
for endless reasons

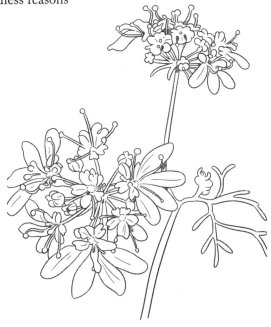

july

a car diffuser is of utmost importance
when road-tripping across country
peppermint oil and a purity blend
promote alertness,
focus transcends
a few drops on a cotton ball in your vents
stimulating concentration sure makes sense
late night driving
eyes widen
forcing them open
heaviness weighs
one more hour to go
don't let them close
coffee refills,
caffeine drinks
oils are essential
mints are preferential
energy needed
patience exceeded
destination ahead
stop dead
you know the feeling
sleep appealing
good night, oils.
you've spoiled, yet again!

if your summer travel requires flying
essential oils are worth applying

peppermint behind each ear relieves the pressure
a drop on the roof of your mouth makes breath fresher
don't worry about the tsa rules
your oils can travel on the plane with you
15 milliliters of pure goodness
is well below the 3-ounce limit

august

summer's ultraviolet rays cause concern
skin reddens, dries and burns
sandalwood oil's cooling properties
calms the burn with healing qualities
it evens tans, removes germs
soothes skin, tightens, firms
anti-inflammatory eucalyptus
numbs the pain a burn can cause us
its mentholated quality
is not to be taken lightly
less is more
it will restore
oils, our summers would be nothing without you!

september

as autumn falls
the trees give way
to the changing leaves
drop, drop
drift away
wind whisks
air chills
multi-colored foliage
new growth
apple-filled trees
pumpkins lined up
bales of hay piled
a season of festivals
harvests, migrations
scarecrow creations
the smells of autumn
waft through the air
oils are essential at this time of year
cinnamon bark essential oil
musky and spicy
extracted from the bark of its tree
supports heart-healthy bodies
fosters good circulation
decreases inflammation
used by ancient egyptians
valued as gold
stories untold
strengthens immunity
infinite opportunities

removes nervous tension
improves memory, brain retention
never disappoints
calms sore muscles and joints
helps metabolic functions
controls allergy dysfunctions
fills my tummy
recipes are yummy
cinnamon bark oil, you spoil me
royally

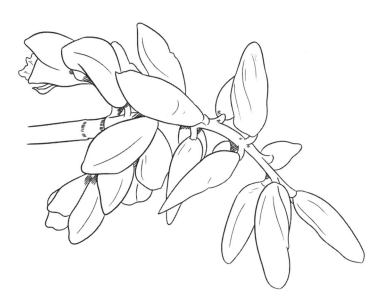

october

spider webs, witches' brew
haunted houses, ghosts and ghouls,
trick or treat, cauldron boils
frankincense is halloween's oil
its mystical power
to heal and fix
blended with any oil
the perfect mix
don't mistake "stein" for "cense"
they're nothing alike
one is frightful,
getting screams
while the other calms the soul
physically, emotionally and all in between
frankincense oil, you spoil us all
winter, spring, summer and fall!

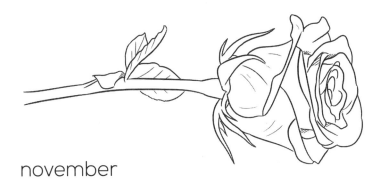

november

ground cools and hardens
leaves cover in full
hibernation
migration
days shorten
preparing for cold weather
as your body makes its way
each day
defenseless in cold
achy joints, running noses
poor circulation increases
cold hands and feet
warm yourself
black pepper is essential
preferential
it's hot and spicy
so please dilute
this oil's power
knows no substitute
gently work

into hands and feet
discomfort obsolete
blood flowing,
heat glowing
immediate warmth
all of the citrus oils
are essential this season
rid germs in the air
boost your immunity
awesome opportunity
to fight infection
build protection
for overall wellness
merits are endless

december

lights flicker in the distance
twinkling as they speak to us
spreading cheer
spreading excitement
it's the holiday season
late night shopping
traffic's bopping
there's a buzz in the air
minds are working
thinking, planning
preparing, inviting
calendars are busting

so much to do
need to energize
feeling pressure rise
emotions recognized
oils, come spoil me
help me cope
the positivity you evoke
in me
understanding what i need
rolled over pressure points
in the hands and feet
breathing in your beauty
supporting me in every way
securing possibilities
pushing me forward
keeping me going
resolute
my oils suit me
refocus me
keep me plodding ahead
knowing what's important here
family gatherings
full bellies
trimming trees, gift giving
togetherness,
festivities,
fir and pine diffusing
reminiscing
holiday wishing
tradition
oils have become an integral part
of traditions
an integral part
of all that i am

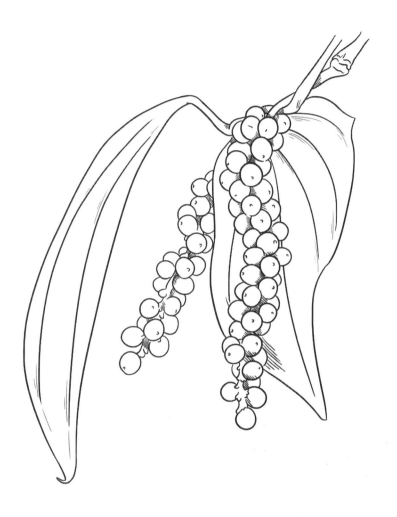

reflecting on my year in oils

reflection is key. reflection enables self-awareness and the ability to consider one's work with a new lens. an honest lens. a lens of objectivity. the truth is, essential oils have become a part of me. the me that's been me for the last 50 years has been changed. changed for the better. these oils enhance my every day as they guide me and support me in every way. upon reflection, this is hard to believe. it's hard to imagine that these oils can inhabit my thoughts and actions the way they do. that each day as i feel and as i think, i consider how my oils can help; how they can bring my family good health; how they can stimulate feelings of bliss, satisfaction and sheer happiness. they can calm our bellies and dull aches and pains. they empower us to learn and find success in all we do. i love that essential oils have infinite possibilities. that there are hundreds to choose from. hundreds of bottles filled with essential scents and essential benefits. that they can be used in so many ways (aromatically, topically, internally, blended, singly, on pressure points, directly on spot, in my diffuser, etc.) as the cycle of life encircles our actions year in and year out, so do essential oils. they are an essential part of each minute, hour, day, month, season and year.

an open letter

dear oils,

i wish i could tell you
all that you mean to me
all that you have brought me
you've empowered me to become a healer
a healer of the mind and body
just like you
you have pushed me to strive for more
to take action instead of choosing passivity
to learn and study about your science
to understand how to safely benefit from you
keeping in mind how strong you truly are
i don't take advantage of your power
i fully appreciate it; each and every day
what are you thinking, oils?
i would love to hear your thoughts
how it feels to be you
knowing how you've changed the lives of so many
how you've fixed them after so many years
how you have transitioned us from helplessness to empowerment
how does that feel to you?
sometimes there are those who doubt you
who call you a phony and a fake
i wish you could shout at the top of your lungs,
"i can help you!"
i wish they could hear it directly from you
only you can defend
you know the facts
if i only had the chance to meet you
to chat
to know what it feels like

to work your way through my body
and encourage it to operate at full capacity
to do what you do
when i mention you to others, do you hear?
do you feel how impassioned i am?
how i trust you completely and fully?
i know that you can't remedy every ailment
and that disease will still strike when our bodies are out of sync
but i do know that you can shorten or lessen an outbreak
that you can suppress symptoms that nag
what else can i expect of you?
nothing.
oils, you must know that i am forever grateful
forever thankful!

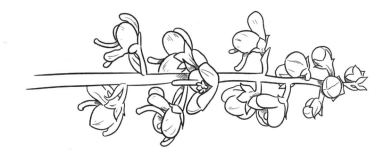

about the author

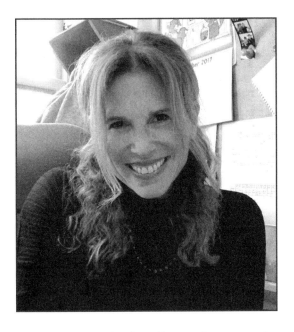

Alysa Beer is an essential oils wellness advocate, wife, mother, and educator for twenty-five-plus years. Alysa has a Bachelors in communications from BU and a Masters in elementary education from NYU. Alysa is dedicated to using essential oils in her daily life.

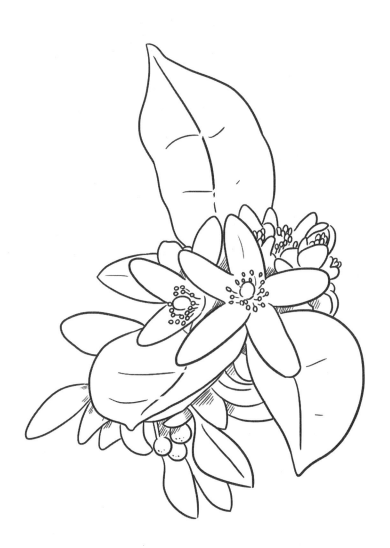